DISCOVER THE PERFECT DIET FOR YOUR PERSONALITY TYPE

OSCAR MENDEZ

Discover the Perfect Diet for Your Personality Type

PERSONALITY

BASED DIETING

TABLE OF CONTENTS

INTRODUCTION

Is your body weighing you down? It could have something to do with your personality. Your personality type influences almost every other aspect of your life. Your career, relationships, and social life are a direct reflection of your personality type. While these aspects have a direct link to personality traits and basic human interaction, research has shown that diet is also one of the core aspects that complement your personality. Dieting often takes a back seat when analyzing personality types. Success in your career can also be traced back to your personality type. Additionally, basic human interaction and relationships have a direct correlation with your personality type.

Research on dieting and health suggests that your personality type will determine your overall health. There are sixteen different types of personalities based on scientific theories of classification. While science would give a better insight on personality traits, when it comes to health and fitness, deriving the most important and relevant factors are necessary for trying to demystify personality traits in relation to dieting and overall health. The following table highlights the most important aspects of daily living in relation to eating patterns and the corresponding personality types. These aspects are fundamental in driving the influence one's personality has to food.

Eating Pattern Personality

- The Late Night Eater Introvert, Quiet, Loner, Reserved
- The Impulsive Eater Spontaneous, Introvert, Perceiver
- The Normal Eater Extrovert, Average, Adaptable, Flexible
- The Extreme Dieter Introvert, Skeptic, Thinker
- The Controlled Grazer Extrovert, Perceiver, Outspoken, Enthusiastic, Planner
- The Travelling Eater Extrovert, Adventurous, Fun Loving

The above personality types cover every eating pattern, from the heavy eater to the extreme dieter. The following study seeks to examine the above popular eating patterns about personality types to come up with the perfect diet plan that complements each particular personality type.

SUMMARY

The Late-Night Eater

The late-night eater is an introvert, but not exactly anti-social. They will normally eat with others but tend to go back for more while everyone else is asleep. Food tastes better at night and tastes even better in bed. They do not mind feeling uncomfortably full before bedtime.

The Impulsive Eater

The impulsive eater is spontaneous when it comes to food. Their introverted personality works well for them, as they do not like being subjects of ridicule when it comes to eating.

They do not follow a regular eating pattern and tend to overindulge when there is plenty of food available.

The Normal Eater

This is the most popular eating pattern. A normal eater is an extrovert, and does not mind eating in groups, as well as eating alone.

They do not attach a preference to either eating alone or in groups. A normal eater can adapt to any food and does not think beyond getting full.

The Extreme Dieter

The extreme dieter is a skeptic when it comes to food. Their abnormal eating patterns trigger withdrawal tendencies because they are introverts. An extreme dieter has a negative attitude towards food and will find it hard to overindulge. If not managed properly, an extreme dieter's fitness regime might turn into a disorder

The Controlled Grazer

The controlled grazer does not attach much thought into the food they eat. Controlled grazers are the working population. Their daily activities are organized and pre-determined. They are not particularly choosy when it comes to food, although they love experimenting. They find it hard to diet, as the love for different things surpasses the need to be selective.

The Travelling Eater

The traveling eater is adventurous by nature, an extrovert and more often than not fun loving. They tend to explore when it comes to food; they find it hard to stick to a diet regime as they spend most of their time on the go.

The Extreme Dieter

They say you are what you eat. What if you do not eat at all? Extreme dieting is gaining pace as far as dieting trends go. The existence of foods that support extreme dieting goes on to prove the popularity of the trend, with the need to starve one's self being an alternative to exercising and fitness regimes. Exercise require lots of patience, discipline and hard work. Extreme dieting is perceived as a faster way to shed off fat. Some cases of extreme dieting end up being full blown eating disorders. Fitness experts and dietitians do not recommend extreme dieting as a fitness plan, as it is unhealthy and unnatural. Recent studies show that four out of ten overweight adults have considered extreme dieting as a fitness plan, with two out of the four implementing the plan.

Extreme dieters are introverts, often battling self-confidence issues. To reveal the psychology behind extreme dieting, establishing the root cause of the problem is congruent to finding a solution. What starts out as healthy intentions turn out to be an extremely unhealthy and ill-advised measure. The problem can be traced back to stress, emotional turmoil, negativity and inconsistent and wrong diet plans.

DIETING AND PERSONALITY TYPES EXPLAINED

EXPLAINED

Eating Patterns, Characteristics, and Facts

An Extreme dieter

- Is ''afraid'' of food. To put this fact into context, food is deemed as their worst enemy regarding various aspects of life, including social, career and mental aspects. This is the reason why models starve themselves and often suffer from Anorexia; a medical eating disorder.
- Lack proper nutrition. As a result, their immune system is weak and they are vulnerable to illnesses and diseases. The white blood cells are weak due to lack of enough nutrients.
- Experience heightened cholesterol levels.

A study in Molecular Psychiatry revealed that anorexics experience genetic mutation that affects the body's ability to process cholesterol. The heart becomes vulnerable to serious health complications, including hypertension and heart attacks.

- Is vulnerable to developing type I diabetes. Low immunity in the body triggers abnormal cell reactions. If the pancreas falls prey to such abnormalities, the body fails to manage insulin production, thus leading to diabetes
- Is always hungry and thirsty. The body is struggling to maintain optimum levels of productivity and functionality, but there is no food to support it. This leads to increased hunger and thirst.
- Suffers from self-esteem issues. An extreme dieter is always uncomfortable around people and is often intimidated by large crowds and social gatherings. They will avoid

confrontation on the issue at all costs.

- Can go to extremes to support their diet regime including self-induced vomiting, taking diet pills and avoiding eateries to reduce temptations.

An Extreme Dieter's Diet Plan

The disadvantages and repercussions of extreme dieting far outweigh the benefits. While the intentions might be deemed as good, going to extremes to lose weight is scientifically proven to border on the dangerous. You risk losing a lot more if you deprive your body of essential nutrients. Forget what you see on TV and/or have read about over the Internet. The 7-day extreme weight loss plans are meant for the desperate and weak minded.

They might work, but you might have to live with permanent damages associated with them.

They will tell you that you'll look great, feel confident and be very elaborate about it. They will leave out the negative technical aspects of such programs; how convenient! The following are tips, dos and don'ts will go a long way to help you achieve total body control and will provide answers to holistic, safe and natural dieting.

Tips

- Start by developing a positive attitude towards food, one bite at a time. Changing your perception towards mealtimes can go a long way in altering what you are doing wrong in terms of dieting.
- Improve your confidence and self-esteem.
- Shy away from negativity.
- Don't start eating immediately. Come up with a progressive plan on your way to normal dieting to avoid the chance of binge eating.
- Start with the end in mind. Develop a plan that fits your schedule perfectly with no need to skip meals or starve yourself.
- Be realistic. Set achievable goals, and stick to them. Losing 60 pounds a week is unrealistic, unsafe and if possible, comes with a price.
- Proper nutrition requires an investment in your overall well-being. Research extensively and consult widely with regard to proper nutrition.

What to do

You are already dieting. You know almost everything there is to know in terms of losing weight. Use the same information to come up with a diet plan that is healthy.

- Make friends. Improve your social life and be around positive, like-minded individuals who can help you change your perception towards healthy dieting

- Pay close attention to your body. Extreme dieting is sometimes ill-informed and unnecessary. Your body is unique in its own way and at times popular dieting regimes may not work for you. Know when to start and stop dieting.

- Answer the following questions. Does your body accumulate weight fast? Is your metabolism rate fast or slow? What are my options when it comes to healthy eating? How does my body respond to dieting?

- Identify foods that you can eat comfortably. Guilt free food groups include fruits and vegetables, high-fiber foods, whole grains and sugar-free foods.

- Get professional advice. Your physician will tell you the truth about extreme dieting and the options you have if you intend to continue using that measure. Extreme dieters are more often than not following an ill-advised fitness regime that proves detrimental health-wise in the end. Opinions

from qualified nutritionists and medical practitioners can
help improve your dieting regimes.

What not to do

- Do not skip meals. Extreme dieting involves starving yourself. There are more psychological effects regarding food deprivation than what the extreme dieter in you knows.
- Do not stop extreme dieting immediately. If you have already started, progression is the key. You are more susceptible to binge eating as a result of switching diets.
- Do not stop exercising. Your body needs time to adjust from extreme dieting to more healthy options.
- Ignore the hype surrounding fast weight loss. The sales pitches might get to you, but do not let them.
- Opt out of diet pills. Supplements should be prescribed. They might say it is natural and safe, but how safe is safe when it comes to your body? Consult professionals on the safest medical treatments available to avoid falling prey to dubious fitness regimes and pills.

When on an extreme diet, you are five times more likely to develop eating disorders, according to recent studies. Properly managing your diet and avoiding extremes can go a long way in improving your general health. Remember, your general wellness is the whole point of dieting. Matching your personality with a safe diet that works is your best weapon against self-deprivation. No self-respecting dietician or nutritionist can accurately incorporate extreme weight loss plans into normal productive living.

THE IMPULSIVE
EATER

I mpulsive eating, otherwise known as compulsive or binge eating is when you just cannot stop having a bite of everything. An impulsive eater is a feeler rather than a thinker, an introvert rather than an extrovert and a perceiver. An impulsive eater does not put much thought into what they choose to devour and is not as social as a regular eater.

Feelings and food go hand in hand and they perceive that the best way to handle stress is by seeking solace in food. An impulsive eater feels powerless when it comes to controlling food intake. On the extreme, impulsive eating is accompanied by feelings of stress, shame, guilt and eventually depression. It develops into a disorder in the latter stages of development.

Impulsive eating is very treatable and natural remedies actually work. Learning to break the cycle goes a long way in reversing impulsive eating tendencies. Developing a healthier relationship with food takes time and with proper training and focus a turn-around is possible. Research has shown that binge eating starts in late puberty and early adulthood.

Eating Patterns, Characteristics and Facts
an Impulsive Eater

- Experiences the inability to stop eating even when not hungry and can continue eating even when full.
- Eats lots of food within a short time period
- On the extreme, an impulsive eater hides food and can wait for as long as it takes to eat when no one is around
- Eats normally when around other people, but gorges down a whole lot more when no one is there to watch or criticize.
- Does not have a scheduled mealtime and will eat whenever the mood strikes any time of the day
- Does not feel comfortable when food is unavailable. An impulsive eater will avoid places or activities that keep them away from food for very long.
- Will stop at nothing to get a plateful of food when appetite kicks in
- Will eat anywhere as long as the food is available. This includes on the street, while traveling, in the office or while partaking of activities such as reading, watching TV or even idling around
- Will eat when stressed, and eat more when the stress goes away.
- Is characterized by feelings of guilt, shame, and embarrassment when taking more than is necessary.
- Can trace back the binge eating habit to social and cultural

risk factors. This includes having a parent who used to or still uses food to comfort or reward their children. The children attach feelings of self-worth and satisfaction to food.

- Psychologically is inclined to attach psychological risk factors to food. Depression is a leading factor that can cause impulsive eating tendencies.
- Feels satisfied both physically and mentally after a heavy eating session. A binge eater finds it hard to stay away from food, no matter the time of day or activity they are undertaking. This includes screen time, working and while socially active.
- Is most happy during holidays when over-eating tends to be justified. The feeling of guilt is suppressed as almost everyone is taking more than is necessary.

An Impulsive Eater's Diet Plan

Impulsive eating is more of a cycle. It can begin at any age of the cycle. A binge eater's pattern cycles around deprivation, an overwhelming urge to devour, then causes binge eating, uncontrolled eating, followed by a diet regime to control the eating patterns, then cycling back to deprivation. Breaking the cycle at manageable and crucial stages is the solution to curing the impulsive eating. Studies show that binge eating is psychologically controlled. The brain has been trained to associate certain feelings with food, and managing involves diverting the brain's function away from food. Breaking the cycle at the deprivation stage is the surest way to control impulsive eating, and the following tips, dos and don'ts could help a binge eater lose weight and manage their health effectively.

Tips

- Identify your weak points. This involves knowing what triggers the urge to eat tons of food at a go.
- Tolerance. It takes a great deal of getting used to living with the urges to eat unnecessarily, especially when on a diet plan.
- Manage your emotions. Is it a shame? Loneliness? Fear? Anxiety? Train yourself to nip the urges before they develop by identifying the feelings that trigger the binge eating tendencies.
- Research. Get to know everything there is to know about binge eating. A lot of it has to do with what you do not know. Do not be afraid to consult an expert in the field for more insight.
- Empower yourself. Stay away from stressful or anxious situations.
- Control all your cravings. All the curveballs life throws your way are a passing cloud. Learning how to deal with them away from food goes a long way to alleviating binge eating.

What to Do

- Start afresh. Get rid of all fatty and sugary foods from your house. Give them away if you can't dispose of them. Turn your fridge green and make your home a healthy haven
- Learn to lose weight while eating. Confusing? It's not. To fully understand the concept behind eating to lose weight, start by making a plan on how to manage bulk eating. Create an astringent and complex extreme plan that is both effective and easy to manage.
- Get rid of sugar and carbs. Sugar cravings are by far the strongest and easiest to succumb to. They follow a chain whereby you start by eating sugary foods, then the need to follow up with fizzy drinks is imminent. That is why soda, fried chicken, and fries are popularly sold as a package.
- Move. Be active. If the store is a few blocks away, wear your training shoes and walk there. Do not stop for a donut on the way, just bring your bottle of water to keep you hydrated.
- Eat clean. Make it standard practice to start with healthy foods before eating carbs. You are good at eating a lot. Fill up on whole grains, vegetables, and sugar-free drinks.
- Whenever the mood strikes, train your mind to go for colorful fruits and vegetables. Get your daily dose of energy from fruits vegetables and whole grains.
- Always include fiber in your diet. Slowly work your way up

to a high fiber content food and ignore the need to spoil yourself.

- Always know what you are eating. Read the labels, ask about the ingredients and to be safe, train yourself to prepare your own meals. This should not be a problem based on your introvert personality.
- Exercise more and sign up for a fitness plan. There is a lot you can gain just by be-ing around people with the same mentality as you. On the extreme, there are support groups you can join for more insight and positivity.

What not to do

- Do not eat alone. Overeating tends to happen when you are all alone and nobody is criticizing your portions.
- Avoid stressful situations if possible. Get a positive outlook on life. If need be, get help and embrace positive criticism with a smile.
- Avoid negativity at all costs.
- Do not give up on foods you love. Take everything in moderation, unless you are planning on a highly restrictive diet plan.
- Do not give up. Healthy eating is a process and anyone can achieve total body control with the right attitude. This might sound cliché, but a healthy heart starts with a healthy mind. It all starts with self-acceptance.
- Do not overthink. This can work against you. Gather a lot of information regarding impulsive eating and filter out the chaff.
- Enough information is what you need.
- Avoid extremes. You are more susceptible to frustrations if extreme dieting does not work.
- Finally, professional care for impulsive eating is highly recommended.

Often individuals experience a positive outcome after seeking professional help. The odds of you improving your health after consulting a professional are high, so take the chance. Make friends who will positively influence your diet regime. Stay away from negativity and always be happy.

The Night Eater

T he night eater prefers to take meals either in bed or in front of the TV. Eating at night is so common you could be developing an eating disorder like the Night Eating Syndrome, without even knowing it. Night eating syndrome is a characteristic of delayed circadian or daily food intake. While people who like eating beside the night lamp overlooking the television feel like they simply have no control over the urges, the consequences are detrimental, to say the least.

Night eating can be traced back to an individual's personality, with introverts and the "couch potatoes" being the most susceptible to night eating patterns. Some cases border on the extreme, with studies showing that depression, substance abuse, and sleeping disorders are leading causes of night eating syndrome

Eating Patterns, Characteristics

and Facts A Night Eater

- Feels like they have no control over the urge to fix something to eat in the middle of the night.
- Will eat almost anything available, with fried food, crisps, popcorns and snacks be-ing the resolute foods of choice
- Has trouble sleeping and prefers falling asleep on the couch with the TV on or the book they are reading close to them
- Will find it hard to form a standard eating pattern, and does not prefer eating in groups. The dinner table is unnecessary as eating is impulsive and they will snack whenever the mood strikes
- Prefers preparing their own food. More often than not, a night eater will make a sandwich when others are asleep. The need to be self-sufficient when it comes to food makes them give up conventional eating methods
- Will have several side dishes after dinner. The leftovers are a darling and they will ''modify'' the available food to satisfy the existing craving at that time
- Loves takeout. The delivery service number is always on speed dial, as cravings could strike any time of the night
- Will experience an increased appetite when it's all dark outside. During the day the eating patterns are normal, but at night the normal eating patterns do not apply. If busy, they will prepare food first, then get to work.

- When out and about at night, they will always find time to grab something to eat even when not hungry
- More often than not accompanies the food with beer, a stimulant or fizzy drinks. Fried food is a favorite and healthy food comes second
- Is not particularly choosy if snacks or pizza slices are unavailable. They will not dismiss greens or fruit, and will more often than not fire up the stove to spice up the flavor.
- Tends to eat more after dinner than at breakfast and lunch combined
- Has trouble falling asleep if they have not had an eating session, and it gets worse if they are feeling hungry without the possibility of eating or snacking until morning.
- Is not particularly happy about their eating urges before bed

A Night Eater Diet Plan

Nutrition experts and health coaches recommend a diet plan designed to alter a night eater's habits and nocturnal eating tendencies for improved health and weight-loss.

Night eaters tend to be overweight, as they eat more when at rest, and when their basal metabolic rate is very low. The following tips are designed to change eating patterns to ensure every bite contributes to overall wellness in pursuit of a healthy lifestyle and a heart friendly personality. If you are a night eater, here are a few tips to get you started, and most importantly, what to do and what not to do.

Tips

- Consider cognitive behavior therapy. The therapy is structured to change your attitude towards nocturnal eating. Studies relating to the subject reveal that the leading cause of night eating disorders has to do with what we tell ourselves. Taking charge of your feelings towards night eating is the basis of corrective measures.
- Get resourceful information from reliable websites, books, and journals on how to change your night experience regarding food.
- If eating at night, avoid anything starchy and as carbohydrates.
- Switch to low-fat food, lean meat, non-fat dressings, and avoid seasoning healthy food.
- Fill up on greens instead of carbs and fizzy drinks.
- Be hydro-friendly. Water may not be a direct substitute for soda, but it can work to reduce your portions

What to do

- Eat during the day. The probability that you will be active during the day is higher than at night. Make sure you do not skip a meal during the day, especially in the morning, to give your body enough time to burn the calories before retiring at night.
- Go out often, and not to a restaurant or drive-thru. Spend more hours away from your bed or couch and TV.
- Switch off the TV, starve yourself of movies. Studies show that you are more likely to want to snack if you have something requiring zero effort to do, including watching the TV or playing board games.
- Be social. More often than not, we find ourselves craving food when all alone and in need of something interesting to do. Also, you are more likely to overeat when no one is watching. Invite friends over or visit. This can go a long way to help you avoid eating at night.
- Be futuristic. Imagine the world where you sleep right, do not wake up in the middle of the night to fix a sandwich, and leave the leftovers for the morning. Positive imagination is known to alter our attitude and the same applies when it comes to food.

What not to do

- Avoid eating alone. When eating in or go-ing out, tag a friend or bring your child along. You will feel uncomfortable ordering more than is reasonable
- Avoid fried food. Carbs are closely associated with the hormone Serotonin that controls our "feel good" emotions.
- Avoid stressful situations. You tend to eat more when stressed. Live a little, and enjoy the pleasures of life away from the frying pan and refrigerator.
- Change associating screen time with food.

Turn on the TV and just watch what is on. If cravings strike, go for low-calorie food and always keep water at an arms-length. Snack in moderation.

- Avoid eating fast. Overweight people eat faster than healthy people. At night, burn more hours with one plate than going for re-fills. It is a simple exercise, but it can dramatically help you lose weight especially if you are nocturnal when it comes to eating.
- Do not eat unnecessarily. If you are already full, go for a glass of water. The discomfort will make you avoid eating.
- Do not starve yourself during the day in the name of losing weight. The suppressed urge to eat reveals itself at night and it can even double up while you are at rest.
- Avoid hearsay and myths. A lot of ideology about dieting and weight-loss exercise is based on poor research and unjustified science.

The science behind digestion while at rest is that your body while at rest requires almost no energy to function. While asleep, your body only needs the energy to keep your vital organs functional, including the circulatory, respiratory and digestive systems. With this in mind, you can schedule eating time accordingly.

The Normal Eater

Y ou probably know someone who never makes an effort to mind what they eat. They will devour almost anything. Medical dietary restrictions do not apply to them. The normal eater is the average citizen, oblivious of dieting and does not feel the need to subscribe to any dieting regime. A normal eater's fridge has a little bit of everything. When the pocket is deep they will spoil themselves and when the ATM card runs dry, they cut down on exotic dining. To put everything into context, the normal eater is mindless, later; neither their waistline nor their chubby cheeks will keep them away from carbs. Normal eaters love meat as much as they love a bowl of salad.

Normal eaters are neither feelers nor judgmental in nature. They are extroverts and process information with no underlying rules. At dinner, they are not exactly choosy and anything on the menu goes. They are, however, mindful of their health and do not overindulge often.

Eating Patterns, Characteristics and Facts

A Normal Eater

- Does not see the need to follow a diet regime. On average, they eat fewer vegetables, oils, fruits, dairy, and poultry
- Will meet or exceed the daily guideline allowance of all foods, but on average they will naturally eat a balanced diet, without the need of follow-up
- They tend to eat more sugars than is recommended and will eat foods high in calories. They, however, naturally compensate for the excessive calorie intake on days when high-calorie foods are out of reach.
- They will settle for anything without the need to go an extra mile to satisfy a craving, unlike night eaters.
- Does not feel the need to be empowered when it comes to food. A normal eater will neither read the diet advisory section on a magazine, nor the recipe page.
- A normal eater might gain weight unknowingly, and will probably slow down on the carbs once their clothes start tightening up.

This, however, does not mean they will entirely stop eating fatty foods.

- Eats whenever the mood strikes. Since they are average consumers, the mood will naturally strike in the morning, at midday or when its dark outside. They, however, are more likely to skip meals, especially if their daily schedule is demanding.
- Do not feel the need to compensate for missed meals highlighting their perception over their feelings or personality.
- Does not attach feelings to food and will not feel offended if their piece of meat is missing from the fridge.
- Will not go an extra mile to satisfy cravings. Most foods are readily available to them, as an average person's taste buds are not that sensitive to specific foods.
- Does not have any dietary restrictions. Since they naturally meet the daily guideline amount, most lifestyle diseases do not catch up with them.
- The fact is, however, some cannot escape packing pounds on eventually, especially if they are not active or do not exercise regularly.

A Normal Eater's Diet Plan

If a normal eater has to transition to a diet, it might take them the time to adjust. Remember, they do not feel the need to eat healthily. What might trigger a diet could be their doctor's orders, external influence or succumbing to the perception that a healthy weight is more desirable. Normal dieters might find it hard to give up normal eating, as all foods are important and temptations take center stage. Once the diet regime is up and running, they might stick to it. The problem is that it takes them time to experience change and more likely than not they will drop the diet, exercise or fitness plan. Here are a few tips on how to successfully manage a diet plan if you are eating normally.

- ***Prepare yourself for success.*** You are probably setting yourself up for failure if you do not prepare adequately. You might end up "cheating on" your new rules regarding food if you take a step overnight or instantaneously
- ***Moderation.*** Slowly train your mind to be content with enough. As you start your diet plan, see the bigger picture in terms of restrictions. Do not entirely scrap your favorite pizza, or hot wings. Do not delete the delivery guy's number from your contact list; just remove it from speed dial
- ***Sugar is your nemesis from now on.*** I am in no way implying that taking sugar is a don't do, but knowing it is not good is enough

- ***Fruits and veggies are your new closest friends.*** If

you have never set foot into a farmer's market, this is the time. The need to overindulge from time to time was there, and it will not go away overnight

- **Fiber.** You probably do not pay close attention to foods rich in fiber. Fiber is good for you. You can eat as much as you want, with no physical consequences.
- **Research.** The more information you have, the more you will feel empowered and there exists tons of useful resources you can utilize, to know more about dieting.

What to do

- *Get in the kitchen.* Prepare your own food to match your diet plan. This is the first and most important step. The healthiest way to ensure you are eating right is by preparing the food yourself. You will also be able to replace unhealthy food with healthier alternatives. Switching from trans-fats to healthy, cholesterol free fats is simpler if you are do-ing it straight from your kitchen.
- *The labels tell a lot.* Be aware of what you eat. Manufacturers say it is healthy and natural, but is it? The composition table is al-ways accurate for anything that has passed standardization.
- *Hydrate.* Water flushes out toxins naturally.

Dehydration brings about tiredness and headaches.

- *Fiber.* Foods rich in fiber are golden. They include oatmeal, brown rice, unprocessed cereal, celery, barley, whole meal bread, tomatoes and most fruits are rich in fiber. Opt for everything unprocessed. Dieting is never easy, as taste is a factor you will have to keep at bay.
- *Calcium.* Include a significant amount of calcium in your diet. Foods rich in calcium include low-fat cheese, milk, sugar-free yogurt, vegetables, and fruits. Almost every other type contains high amounts of calcium including black beans, pinto beans, and black-eyed peas.
- *Protein.* Eat lots of fish, lean meat, chicken, soy-based products, tofu, nuts, and seeds.
- *Fats.* Contrary to popular belief, not all fats are unhealthy. There are good fats and bad fats. Good fats contribute to a healthy you, while bad fats, especially trans fats, are highly detrimental to a healthy heart.

What not to do

Do not ban certain foods you used to love.

They might be unhealthy, but thinking of them as off-limits could work against you in the long-run. Encourage yourself to diet even more by spoiling yourself in moderation. Do everything you used to, but cut down for the sake of your dieting regime.

- *Stop eating.* When you feel full, stop eating and open that bottled water. That extra spoonful is how it all starts.
- *Avoid fizzy drinks.* If you are going fizzy, make it a diet.
- *Avoid eating out.* Gravy, salad dressings, soup, and sauce may contain high amounts of either sugar or salt. These are bad for you. Order them on-the-side instead. Little changes go a long way in the long run.
- *Do not overindulge in processed snacks.* Instead opt for healthier alternatives. Almost every other snack has a healthier alternative.
- Anything packaged or canned contain hidden fats, even when the label reads "healthy."
- The normal eater's secret to a successful diet regime is moderation. While giving up on certain, foods including deep fried foods, candy, and processed food is not an option, cutting down and alternating with healthier options is the best way to win when it comes to dieting.

The Travelling Eater

G ranted, keeping up with a diet regime while on the road could be as daunting as traveling itself. You are constantly on the move, with no time to exercise or be choosy about what you eat. It requires next-level discipline to stay fit. Weight-wise, it could go either way. You might find yourself either gaining or losing weight. Either way, traveling will take a toll on your health. Where will you prepare your healthy snack? Truck drivers, business travelers, and leisure tourists find it hard to maintain a fitness regime. The restaurant or drive-thru at the gas station will more likely than not be selling everything to go. People tend to eat more while traveling than on the job, lazing around the house or working in an office combined.

Starving yourself is not an option; you need the energy to remain efficient throughout the day. Not enough water in the world can replace food. The traveler has an adventurous, outgoing personality. The love for experimentation is admissible, thus the need to try out different things. When not monitored closely, your personality could be detrimental to your health.

Eating Patterns, Characteristics and Facts

A TRAVELLER

- Is more susceptible to weight gain, scientifically. A recent publication by Cell Magazine revealed a link between switching time zones and weight gain. Scientists studied the behavior of the bacteria Mi-crime that thrives in the stomach. The study involved two people traveling from the USA to Israel. The bacteria had mutated, supporting weight gain and the risk of developing diabetes.

- Will more likely than not eat unhealthy due to limitations. While on a flight, for example, your choices are limited, especially if you are not flying first class. Truckers will most likely end up having a burger, coke, and fries during their several pit stops. If you are on a safari for example, you want to feel liberated, so chances are you will over-indulge a little.

- Will struggle to stay hydrated. While on the road, bathroom breaks are disruptive and inconvenient. A traveler would prefer not taking water than having to stop several times to take a number one.

- Finds it hard to eat healthily. Who has time to visit the farmer's market when constantly on the road? Easy, to-go foods are the easiest option. This could lead to more than ideal sugar intake that goes straight to the waistline.

- Does not follow a constant eating pattern. The variables are alternating faster than our ability to control them with regard to food. If you are a cross-state or an international traveler, you would have to eat what you can get. Lack of information about what you eat could be working against your weight management endeavor.

- Might have no choice but to overeat. So, you are planning a trip to Asia, you think your options when it comes to food are wide? Think again. Asians love cholesterol, they just cannot have enough of deep fried everything! It's not the sushi that will get to you; it's the side dishes and accompaniments. The fries on the side will go straight to your hips. What's more? You cannot leave food on your plate unfinished, it is deemed offensive.

- Is simply exhausted. Fighting off exhaustion involves eating food rich in energy, or just going hard and drinking a can of energy drink. Foods and drinks rich in energy are only harmless if you actually utilize all the energy in them. If it happens when you are at rest, the glucose is stored underneath your skin as fat. Since you are constantly on the move, you might not experience the adverse effects of glucose. But what if you are a "bus potato" and all your movement is automotive related? Two words, weight gain.

A Traveller's Diet Plan

It requires a great deal of discipline to stay healthy while constantly on the move. Your best bet would be to go the extra mile to avoid gaining unhealthy weight. The weather, the food itself and your schedule all work against your fitness regime. You would need to counter all the adverse effects of these variables and come up with a system you can follow. The following tips, dos and don'ts can go a long way to alleviating weight gain.

Tips on making smart food choices on the road

- Always be packing. Carry your own food while flying or traveling by road. You will lose the need to spend extra on unhealthy snacks. Predetermine your breakfast, lunch, and dinner and if it is not too much trouble, pack it and move along with it.
- Eat a heavy breakfast. Include foods rich in energy on your breakfast menu. Opt for fruits and vegetables for lunch and supper. As we mentioned earlier, it takes a great deal of discipline to remain healthy on the go.
- Reward yourself. Never be uptight about trying out local cuisines. The trick is to take everything in moderation. Count your calories if you have to, just don't overindulge
- Wear your training shoes everywhere if appropriate. Always ensure your shoes are as comfortable as possible. This will encourage you to walk more and avoid fatigue. Walk everywhere if possible.
- Hydrate. Your water bottle is your closest friend if you are to maintain optimal weight.
- Got an extra hour to burn? Relax and take a nap. Studies show relaxing your brain while active reduces the chances of cortisol production. Cortisol, the stress hormone, contributes a great deal to weight gain. When you are relaxed, the enemy within will not attack.

What to Do

- ***Locate the nearest farmer's market.*** Take time off your busy schedule and shop for whole foods and fruits. You will not only be aware of what you are eating, you will also put a smile on the face of the locals.
- ***Ask.*** Ask exactly what is in the salad, stew, soup or any other food you are skeptical of. There is no harm in asking, nowhere in the world will you find a sign in a restaurant saying "do not ask about what is on your plate."

Before ordering that dish you have never tried before, politely get to know the contents. If it so happens you like the dish, it might be healthy enough to overindulge and the experience could turn out unforgettable.

- ***Take every chance you get to eat healthily.*** Your next stop might be a fast food restaurant, thus limiting your choices. Do not ignore the grocery store you see next, it might be the only one you come across for the rest of your journey.
- ***Proteins. Lean meat, fish, and beans are great amino acids sources.*** Proteins will stabilize your body's energy needs, and go a long way to improve your concentration and prevent energy lags.

- ***Avoid "feel bad" foods.*** They include carbohydrates, glycemic foods, refined sugars, deep fried food, artificial sweeteners and anything baked and packaged.
- ***Avoid excess alcohol.*** Your efficiency is your best option when it comes to working and traveling. Taking in regular and moderate points here and there is okay, but binge drinking will make you veer off the diet lane.
- ***Fear the unknown.*** If you find it uncomfortable asking what is on your plate, do not feel obliged to eat the food anyway. Visit the farmer's market; eat fruits on the go, if no healthy eatery is available.
- ***Don't skip a meal.*** You will have to compensate later in somewhat unhealthy ways. Carry packed food if lunch or dinner locations are unlikely to be found.

It is a fact that you will most likely than not end up eating unhealthily while on the road. Do research everything you need to know about your trip, including your dieting options. Always be ready to go while dieting on the road, and lower your adventurous personality radar food-wise. Most importantly, have fun; eat everything, but in moderation, and focus on the healthy foods more. Your traveling should not weigh you down.

The Controlled Grazer

The Unguided Grazer does not think about food very much. They will neither make an effort to look for food nor schedule time to eat. The controlled grazer eats at will, more often than not skipping important meals, including breakfast and lunch. They can even go hungry the whole day and eat if the food is conveniently at an arm's length. Their favorite eating joint is in front of the computer, in the office or beside the food truck down the street. The controlled grazer is the career person deeply buried in work and rarely finding time to take a snack.

The controlled grazer finds it very hard to keep track of portions because their eating patterns are irregular, spontaneous and often forced. They might fill up on junk food on the way home from the office or take an occasional bite of an apple at the office. There is simply no telling what they will eat or when, so planning a diet can be one of the hardest things a controlled grazer would have to do.

Eating Patterns Characteristics and Facts

A Controlled Grazer;

- Does not schedule eating time. A controlled Grazer will not stop doing a task to eat. Food is secondary to work and they only eat when it's very convenient for them.
- Does not follow a particular eating trend. The ever busy controlled grazer needs to remember to eat and is not particularly choosy of what exactly to order at the fast food joint or tier one restaurant.
- Tends to eat when hungry. A controlled grazer will feel the urge to eat after prolonged hours without food. They might have a bite in the morning and then grab a heavy takeout meal at 11 PM on the way home.

There is simply no set schedule.

- Is very spontaneous when it comes to food. A controlled grazer is not particularly choosy over what to eat. They do not feel the urge to be choosy and cravings play a huge part in determining what they will devour.

Controlled Grazer Diet Plan

Dieticians and nutritionists have come up with the most effective dietary plan for the working person. The diet is structured to fit into the work schedule of a spontaneous, irregular person, with flexibility in eating patterns being the most important factor.

Tips

- Since there is barely enough time to make a healthy dinner in the kitchen, a healthy takeout should be ideal.
- Consider buying breakfast and lunch in advance. You are more likely to open the lunch pack if it's at an arm's length, than at the canteen on the ground floor of the building you work in.
- Include snacking in your daily "to do" list if you are good at following a laid out schedule.
- Find an already laid out diet plan from a reliable source, maybe the Internet or resourceful articles instead of doing the hard work yourself.
- Do not starve yourself. The body stores fat for this exact function. Your metabolism will slow down if the body is constantly subjected to food deprivation.
- For breakfast consider having energy rich foods including wholemeal bread, low-fat yogurt, skimmed milk, cereal, oatmeal and fiber rich foods. Fruits are also ideal, you can have a plateful of fruit salad or fresh juice, alongside your normal cup of coffee
- If your work entails sitting all day long, snack away! Just keep everything low fat and in small servings. Savory snacks, peanuts, crisps, and cookies can work to excite your taste buds and make up for the restrictive diet you are on Consider filling up on veggies, especially at night. Of all food types, vegetables contain the least amount of sugar, even

lower than fruits.

Controlled grazers enjoy feeling in control of the world around them. The organization takes center stage and the need to organize everything comes naturally. Eating takes a back seat, as their jobs are the most import-ant aspect of their lives. Dieting plans for a controlled grazer need to fit into their work schedule. They would rather skip meals to remain in control of their work, than spend time focusing on their weight. The working mom will sign up for a fitness regime that is prescheduled to not interfere with their work.

The corporate dad will work out or diet within their work schedule and instead of being inconsistent; they would rather seek alternatives to healthy living instead of dieting. That is all part of remaining in control of their working schedule.

What to Do

- If you happen to be a workaholic, or your job demands extensive hours with minimum breaks, dieting could be the least of your worries. Whether working in a hospital, school, on the road always or in the office, your job can take a toll on your weight.
- Your waistline could be taking hits without you knowing, and by the time you realize it and you are uncomfortable with your looks, it's too late. You cannot place blame on your inability to control what happens between 8 am and 5 pm, especially if you have to squeeze in parental duties somewhere along the way.
- After a hard day's work, the kitchen is the last place you would want to end up. Preparing a healthy dinner can seem far out of reach and this is a fact.
- Dieting would be your best option as a controlled grazer if you want to shed those extra pounds. The gym is just not an option, however good the sales pitch is of fitness trainers. However, if you have access to a fitness gym at the workplace it could be an added fitness benefit.
- During the weekends and holidays, be active. Go swimming with friends. The park is also an option if you have little ones. If the distance is reasonable, walk there instead of driving. The little things you do to keep active add up in the long run.

What NOT To Do

Remember, you are trying to lose weight as a controlled grazer. Everything you were doing bordered on the impulsive. The following don'ts can help you maintain your diet and eventually fitness.

- Avoid piling up the carbs while not being physically active. Comfort eating could be your gateway to obesity. Eat everything in moderation, if you cannot stop completely.
- Avoid work-related stress. The stress hormone cortisol is known to trigger fat and sugar cravings and you might end up in fast food restaurants more often than necessary.
- Avoid pulling all-nighters and working late.

Depriving your body of sleep could add to your already existing weight worries. Thanks to the food you will eat during the extra hours of work, you are more likely to gain weight more so than someone who gets eight hours of sleep.

- Stay away from the candy jar, the vending machine, and refrigerator. You might want to reward yourself with a free donut or chocolate bar, but these will act against your weight loss plan.
- Avoid eating in groups. While this might sound off-putting, research has shown that if the person you are eating with orders high-fat food, you are more likely to do the same. If you cannot make them order a bowl of fruit salad like yours,

find other ways to bond with your colleagues. Remember, you are gaining weight because you are a controlled grazer, and a turn-around is necessary.

- ***While at work, avoid sitting for long hours.*** Get those copies yourself, or reorganize the shelves on your own. Take the stairs once in a while and instead of calling a colleague, walk to their office if it makes sense to do so. These small adjustments can add up in the long run.
- If you travel a lot, the wining and dining during business trips can divert your attention from your weight loss plan. Come up with a way to counter this. It could be by drinking a lot of water before meals, filling up on veggies or avoiding alcoholic beverages; as one tends to eat a lot while pouring down the good stuff.

Useful Facts about Dieting - Demystifying Dieting

Myth: Late night eating leads to weight gain.

Fact: Studies by Cambridge University Human Research Center showed that people who ate late at night would burn the same amount of fat as people who ate at lunchtime.

Myth: People struggling to lose weight have a low metabolism.

Fact: No one obese person has been proven to have lower than normal metabolism. Studies have confirmed that overweight people have a faster metabolism rate to compensate for the high food intake.

Myth: Dieting improves one's efficiency and general work rate.

Fact: Studies show that dieting actually dulls the mind, thus leading to reduced productivity. A reduction in brain memory capacity interferes with optimum brain functionality.

Myth: Obesity is linked to one's genes

Fact: Studies show that obesity is 1% genetic and 99% sedentary lifestyle.

Myth: Yogurt helps burn fat

Fact: The fat content in yogurt is almost equal to that in ice-cream. Greek yogurt, for example, contains 10% fat. Artificial sweeteners make matters even worse.

Myth: The ''apple a day keep the doctors away'' slogan is true.

Fact: Compared to tropical foods, fruits such as apples contain traces of carbohydrates that have a low glycemic index and act to slightly raise blood sugar levels. So, mangoes and pineapples will reduce chances of visiting the doctor more so than apples.

Myth: Calories from carbohydrates are healthier than calories from fats.

Fact: Calories from wheat will equally make you as fat as calories from butter.

Myth: Your body shape can be changed by dieting.

Fact: Dieting will trim your body evenly and proportionally. The only way to change your body shape is by designing your exercise regimes to focus on specific areas of your body, for example, do squats to enhance your bum.

Myth: Weight gain is closely related to wheat intolerance

Fact: The numbers are not enough to support the theory. Only 0.1% of overweight people suffer from wheat intolerance.

Myth: Canned fruits and vegetables contain lesser vitamins and nutrients than fresh ones.

Fact: Canned fruits and vegetables are carefully chosen and packed within hours of picking. Furthermore, fresh fruit and vegetables lose significant percentages of vitamins and nutrients during transport and storage.

Myth: Red meat is unhealthy and contributes to weight gain.

Fact: Thanks to improved methods of trimming fats from meat, there has been a significant drop in the fat content in red meat.

Myth: Honey is healthier than sugar.

Fact: Honey contains simple sugars; 75% sugar and 25% water to be precise. A teaspoonful of honey contains 25 calories, while the same amount of sugar contains 16 calories. Honey is a known cause of teeth browning and decay.

Myth: When eating out opt for salads.

Fact: Salad dressings contain more calories than fries and steak. Popular ingredients like mayonnaise, crispy bacon and croutons are high in fats and sugars.

Vital Statistics on Dieting

1. Only one in three children is physically active. Technology has made going out to play unnecessary, with children opting to derive fun from electronics, including gaming consoles, smartphones, and computers

2. 95% of adults do not partake in physical exercises and fitness routines for more than 30 minutes a day. Fitness experts, on the other hand, recommend at least 30 minutes of exercise a day.

3. Children nowadays spend an average of 6 hours a day in front of a screen. This includes phones, televisions, and computers.

4. Since the 1970s fast food restaurants have more than doubled in numbers worldwide, with most successful fast food chains going international. The growth has been attributed to the fact that fast foods are significantly cheaper than whole foods. Takeout is also contributing to the rise in numbers of fast foods worldwide.

5. In 2008, statistics from the World Food Program revealed that close to 50 million people, including over 16 million children, experienced food insecurity.

6. Up to 50% of women have gone through a diet plan at some point in their lives.

7. America is leading in terms of cash spent on dieting and surgical procedures to reduce weight. The numbers are on a

steady increase and are set to rise from the current $53 million as of 2016.

8. Adults in the United States eat an extra 1,100mg of salt a day; with the average consumption currently at 3,400mg and the daily guideline allowance standing at 2,300mg.

9. There is a 70% chance that an overweight adolescent will become obese at adulthood.

10. Health issues related to obesity including chronic diseases, death, and disability require over $200 billion in funding and managing.

Dieting and Healthy Eating, Is There A Difference?

The government is currently measuring the BMI of students. This move is aimed at trying to come up with solutions to weight management right from childhood as they transition into adulthood. Establishing a healthy eating regime or dieting are two ways to naturally lose weight. While the two are closely related, there is a difference between healthy eating and dieting. In the following excerpt, we examine the difference between the two.

Healthy eating is a lifestyle, while dieting is a deviation from normal eating to lose weight. Healthy eating involves optimizing your body by only eating foods that contribute to overall wellness and health. Dieting starts with an end in mind. Giving up foods that are known to contribute to weight gain is the foundation of dieting.

FOODS THAT IMPROVE METABOLISM

There are foods that are scientifically proven to dramatically improve metabolism. These foods should be included in a functional and effective fitness and diet plan.

1. **Almonds.** Almonds contain essential fatty acids known to improve metabolism.
2. **Beans.** All types of beans contain the basic building blocks for optimum metabolism.
3. **Fruits.** The fiber and useful carbs act as metabolism boosters. You can eat as much as you want to enhance digestion and metabolism.
4. **Celery.** In addition to having almost zero calorie content, celery acts to boost your metabolism and breakdown of other foods
5. **Chia.** Chia seeds are rich in metabolism boosting omega -3 fats, fiber, and protein. The combination is a powerful metabolism booster.
6. **Chocolate.** The cacao in chocolate improves your metabolism rate. You should, however, not overindulge to derive its full benefits.
7. **Apple Cider Vinegar.** Mix your apple cider vinegar with lemon juice for your daily dose of metabolism booster.
8. **Cinnamon.** In addition to boosting your metabolism, cinnamon helps manage carbohydrate and sugar cravings.
9. **Coconut oil.** Add coconut oil to your brown rice for a faster and more efficient metabolism.
10. **Coffee.** High-grade coffee is rich in caffeine, which acts to light up your day and improve metabolism therein,
11. **Curry.** There is no better spice to include in your healthy dinner than curry. It will add flavor and act as a metabolism

booster. A win-win.

12. **Fish.** Fish is a great source of protein. The omega 3 oils also act to boost metabolism.

13. **Grapefruit.** The fruit is golden when it comes to dieting. It has been linked to lower insulin levels and boosts metabolism.

14. **Green tea.** The catechin epigallocatechin gallate in green tea is an invaluable immune, metabolism and energy booster.

15. **Seaweed and Seafood.** This combination triggers production of the thyroid hormone, which is a great metabolism enhancer.

16. **Leafy greens.** Kales, spinach and all other leafy greens are known to enhance the burning of fat, especially while exercising.

17. **Watermelon.** In addition to hydration, watermelon acts to improve your metabolism. A slice of watermelon contains enough of the amino acid Arginine that it aids in weight loss.

For the sake of completeness, though it is not food, water enhances both digestion and metabolism, according to a report published in the Journal of Clinical Endocrinology.

WHAT INDUSTRY EXPERTS HAVE TO SAY ABOUT PERSONALITY BASED DIETING

Biggest Loser's Jen Widerstrom in her book

"Diet Right for Your Personality Type" explained how dieting and personality go hand in hand. The fitness trainer went on to elucidate that, "when you do not synchronize your dieting with your personality you, are set for failure." In her book, the author highlights the need for fitness trainers to get to know all about their clients' personality traits before signing them up for a fitness regime. „Most fitness coaches will set you up on a random dieting plan, unaware that the regime does not fit into your behavioral responses to different situations, including food intake. An ineffective and non-functioning diet ends up being frustrating."

Kerri-Ann Jennings MS., RD, a registered dietitian, and author at Eatwell Magazine explains why you need a diet plan that suits your personality. She goes on to give an ex-ample that if a diet plan involves cooking your own meals including breakfast, lunch, and dinner, and you hate being in the kitchen, you are being set up for failure. Your personality includes what you love doing, how you handle situations and how you relate to others. Same goes for food. Having a diet plan that lines up with these factors is the first step to a functioning diet plan.

Dr. Robert Kushner, a fitness expert, professional consultant, and author believes that personality and dieting are the missing links regarding weight loss and healthy living. He goes on to explain that the food we eat has a direct relationship with our attitude towards life in general. Since food impacts our approach to daily living, we can fit our dieting regime to match our lifestyle to ensure our diet plans bring out the best in us with no negative after-effects. Assimilating our diet plans with our personality types improves the ability to maintain a diet plan long enough to reap the benefits. The ''one size fits all'' analogy is misleading, misguided and injudicious.

Dr. Mark Eisenberg from the Jewish General

Hospital in Montreal cited the need for a consistent diet regime. In order to maintain consistency, one has to factor in their interests, behavior patterns and externality influence in their lives. He goes on to say that the majority of people lose a significant amount of weight on average each year. The weight is, however, regained again later. Consistency in dieting is key, as most dieters end up deviating from the norm, hiding behind the need to "reward" themselves.

A study conducted by the National Weight Control Registry sought to investigate the influence of behavior patterns, traits, and habits of dieters. The study collected data through questionnaires from 10,000 individuals who shed over 30 pounds in a calendar year. The study revealed that those who were able to trim over 30 pounds had one thing in common. Their diet plan was unique and tailored to fit into every aspect of their lives. These aspects included family, work, and recreation. Of the 10,000 subjects, those who successfully managed to maintain a healthy lifestyle owed their success to consistency in dieting.

The National Weight Control Registry derives its research from already functioning people instead of random data collection. The already successful people have already proven the practicability of the diet they use. The accurate statistics go a long way in determining what works and what does not.

The registry does not use random focus groups to identify who loses weight eventually. One key research finding revealed that people who successfully manages their weight identified what motivates them and what inhibited their weight loss regime.

Another important research finding led by Harvard Professor Dr. Matthew Gillman from the Obesity Prevention Program revealed that people who start dieting with the end in mind tend to be more effective. Result based dieting focuses on setting realistic and resolute goals. Setting the goals prior to the commencement of a diet plan prevents frustrations and incomplete dieting. Dr. Maria Collazo-Clavell from Mayo Obesity Clinic identified one reason behind unsuccessful weight loss programs is thinking of a short-term diet plan. Examples of short-term diet plans include losing weight for a function, to shed off holiday weight or even to fit into a wedding gown. The people who diet on a short-term basis end up developing very negative attitudes towards fitness programs.

Conclusion

I really want to thank you for reading this book.

I sincerely hope have you received value from it. If you receive value from this book, then I'd like to ask you for a favor, would you be kind enough to leave a feedback for this book on amazon?

<u>Click here to leave a review for this book on Amazon!</u>

Bonus!

wouldn't be nice to know when Amazon's top kindle books go on Free Promotion ? well now it's your chance!!

100 free!!

<u>Click here for Instant Access!!!!</u>

Simply as a thank you for downloading this book ,I would like to give you full Access to an exclusive services that will email you when Amazon's top Kindle books go on free promotion ,If you are someone who is interested in saving a lot of money ,than simply click the link for instant Access !!

www.ingramcontent.com/pod-product-compliance
Lightning Source LLC
Chambersburg PA
CBHW060755260726
48660CB00002B/632